MW00775386

The Portable
Miracle Ball Method

The Portable
Miracle

relieve your pain
reduce your stress

Ball Method

by **Elaine Petrone**

Workman Publishing, New York

Library of Congress Cataloging-in-Publication data is available.

ISBN-13: 978-0-7611-4382-6; ISBN-10: 0-7611-4382-3

Design by Paul Hanson and Paul Gamarello

Workman books are available at special discounts when purchased in bulk
for premiums and sales promotions as well as for fund-raising or educational use.
Special editions can also be created to specification. For details, contact the
Special Sales Director at the address below.

Workman Publishing Company, Inc.
225 Varick Street
New York, NY 10014-4381
www.workman.com

Printed in China
First printing December 2006
10 9 8 7 6 5 4 3 2 1

Dedicated to John, Lucas, and Rose

Praise for
The Miracle Ball Method

"Not only are your Miracle Balls great the way the book advises using them, but I carry one with me—in a little drawstring bag—and use it behind my back when I ride in the car for long periods. I also slip one behind my tailbone when I'm working for long periods at the computer. It really helps my 72-year-old back. Thanks!" —NANCY J.

"Thank you so much for developing the *Miracle Ball Method!* . . . I just can't tell you how much better I feel! I can breathe better too! I really do thank you!" —JEANNA A.

"I have had debilitating chronic neck and back pain for years. . . . Last week I purchased *The Miracle Ball Method,* thinking, 'What have I got to lose?' I was amazed: The first time I used the balls my pain subsided. Nothing else has helped like these balls. Thank you, Elaine, for such a wonderful system, and for making it so simple to use. I am regaining a quality of life I have not had in years." —BARBARA N.

"Thank you for such a simple but highly effective therapy!" —GEORGENA B.

"It has only been about 2 weeks, and I am now almost entirely pain-free. Your ball therapy really is truly a miracle. . . . Thank you, thank you, thank you!" —WENDY B.

Contents

PART ONE

The Basics

PART TWO

On the Ball

Introduction

Welcome to *The Portable Miracle Ball Method*. You may have come to this book looking for relief from pain. You may be looking for a way to ease stress and anxiety. Or you may already be familiar with *The Miracle Ball Method* and be looking for more ways to improve the overall condition of your body. *The Portable Miracle Ball Method* is a book and program designed to offer you relief from whatever ails you in a convenient, small package. *The Miracle Ball Method* is great when you are in the space and privacy of your own home, while *The Portable Miracle Ball Method* is designed to go with you on the road. You can use it at the office, on a plane, in your hotel room, or any of the other places you go, to ensure that you always have energy, feel good, and are able to participate in life to its fullest.

My first book, *The Miracle Ball Method,* was published in 2003, and the response to it was overwhelming. Thousands of readers from around the world contacted me to let me know that using the balls with the method helped relieve the symptoms of back and joint pain, sciatic pain, sleeplessness, rotator cuff problems, headaches, pain resulting from accidents—the list seems endless. I heard from a mother of four who had been suffering since an injury in high school. She told me that after just a few sessions with the Miracle Balls she was almost entirely pain-free. A flight attendant from a major airline wrote to say that she had been using the program to undo the stresses of being on her feet all day. A painter told me that his carpal tunnel syndrome was much better after using the balls. And so on. Fans of the method are astonished to discover that just a few hours or days or weeks of using the balls can ease years of suffering that standard therapies have been unable to address.

I noticed that many of the people who had found relief in *The Miracle Ball Method* were using the balls when they traveled. Some asked me for exercises specific to the ailments and conditions of travel. Others simply raved that the balls helped them stay healthy and sane on long or challenging trips. The idea for *The Portable Miracle Ball Method* was born.

My Story

The *Miracle Ball Method,* for those of you who are new to it, is a therapy that I developed to heal myself after an injury. I was a serious dancer in college and experienced a back injury that became a leg injury that became so serious it ended my hopes of becoming a professional dancer. I went from doctors to chiropractors to physical therapists to other professionals, with no results. My right leg eventually shriveled to half its size, and doctors told me I would never walk without a limp. This was unacceptable to me. I sought alternative opinions, and I met bodywork people who thought differently from the doctors. While some doctors told me to stop moving, some teachers I found told me to keep moving. While most doctors believed I needed to build up my strength, I realized that it wasn't weakness in my body that was causing the pain, but the opposite: My muscles were overworked and their excess tension was the root of my chronic pain. I visited some teachers who worked with balls, some who focused on breathing, and others who worked to realign the body. I absorbed all that they taught me and ended up understanding how to let my body heal itself. The system I created is explained in *The Miracle Ball Method*.

It's been thirty years since my original injury, and, thanks to the Miracle Ball Method, I've found myself in better shape after my injury than I had been before it. These techniques changed my life, and now I have dedicated myself to teaching students and certifying teachers of the method, so that others may benefit from the system as I have.

What is The Miracle Ball Method?

The Miracle Ball Method is deceptively simple. You place a ball under a part of your body, notice your breath, and let your weight be absorbed by the ball. Eventually, your muscles release their tension and the cycle of pain is interrupted.

Pain, no matter what its origin—an injury, stress, alignment problem (for example, scoliosis or poor posture), or perhaps all three—causes excess muscle tension. Let's say you experience an injury. Your muscles tighten up, your breathing becomes less effective, and less oxygen gets circulated to the muscles, so they get even tighter. A cycle of pain has started. Muscles that get tight lose feeling; this makes it difficult for our nervous system to receive feedback from the muscles, and our natural alignment system fails. After a while, all we can feel is the pain without knowing where it comes from. At that point, it's difficult to know where to begin to solve the problem. Also, the whole body is usually affected by an injury. Although you may have hurt your knee initially, when you start to limp you may end up feeling the pain in your back, your shoulders, your neck. Eventually, your whole body is subjected to the problem. The cycle of pain continues until you can find a way to relieve your unyielding muscles.

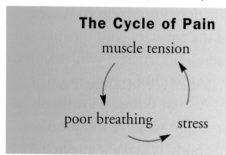

The Cycle of Pain

muscle tension

poor breathing

stress

Excess muscle tension blocks your body's natural alignment system. It makes you inflexible and unresponsive. In my previous book I offer the image of a tennis ball to illustrate this. Imagine gripping a tennis ball in your hand as tightly as you can for hours or even days. First you would experience pain, then after a while your body would adjust and you might stop feeling anything at all. If you removed the ball from your hand, what would happen? Your hand would likely remain in a claw shape for a very long time. Most of us are holding so much tension in our muscles that, despite pain and stiffness, we are unable to relax them: Our bodies have forgotten how. My method is devoted to getting you out of your *thinking body* and developing a dialogue with your *feeling body.* Once you can feel your body, your muscles will be able to relax, and once they can relax, your circulation improves, your breathing returns, and your body can realign itself. *Relief of excess muscle tension equals relief of pain.*

In addition to pain relief, my method offers relief from anxiety and the reshaping of your entire body. You are less likely to feel stressed out when your breathing is deep and easy and your muscles are not clenched. When oxygen flows to tight muscles, those muscles become long and lean and supple. You will see the changes in your body as well as in your mood.

Why the Portable Program?

The *Portable Miracle Ball Method* offers the same relief as the original program, but with the convenience of one small ball instead of two. The ball placements, with a few exceptions, are all new and created for the unique stresses of being on the road. Readers of my first book will notice two or three whole body moves that are essential to any Miracle Ball program (such as the "S" Sound and Standing Body Hang Over), but even these have been enhanced for this new project—for the conditions of travel and being away from home.

Traveling is as stressful as it is exhilarating. The crowded airports, the long lines, the unfamiliar settings, the rushed schedules, the packed commuter trains. Business travelers face even more stress as they deal with work and travel at the same time. When we are not traveling, many of us are at the office, where we are subjecting ourselves to many of the same stresses as we do when we are traveling. We are locked into a fixed position (usually in front of a computer screen or at a conference table), seated in an uncomfortable chair, and often engaged in a repetitive task that can cause stress injuries. We are under deadlines, feeling pressure, and we don't take care of our bodies properly. We hunch over the keyboard, we tuck the phone awkwardly against our neck, and we breathe in a shallow, rushed fashion. All this can exacerbate existing imbalances and create new ones. *The Miracle Ball Method* is the perfect antidote to these problems, but when you are traveling the balls can be cumbersome, hence *The Portable Miracle*

Ball Method. If you are one of the harried, a busy traveler, a stressed-out worker, then welcome. I have created *The Portable Miracle Ball Method* just for you.

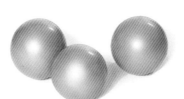

PART ONE

The Basics

CHAPTER ONE

How to Use This Book

The *Portable Miracle Ball Method* works in the same way that the original *Miracle Ball Method* does: It enables you to feel your body, and in turn it enables your body to realign itself. Let's take a moment to see how it works in greater detail.

First, realize that you all you need to get started is the ball and this book. You don't need equipment or a lot of space or different clothing. Some ball placements, especially those done lying down, are more enjoyable in loose-fitting clothing, but the idea is that you take your body everywhere. And you need to *stop holding your breath* wherever you are, whatever you are doing.

Maybe you have one minute. Maybe you have five minutes. Maybe you have more time. If you have only one minute, you'll still get relief. But if you are short on time remember that you still need to follow the directions carefully. You are better off doing one exercise (or one part of one exercise) properly than trying to rush through several.

Here is how I hope you will follow the program and get on the ball. First, focus on beginning your Body Dialogue. When we are in pain or under stress or rushed, lots of times we don't notice our bodies. We don't realize we have shoulders hunched up to our ears, our knees locked, and our hips rotated inward. The only time many of us do notice our bodies is when we experience pain. Pain is your body's way of telling you that you need to make an adjustment. However, most of us at that point are unable to let our bodies self-adjust; we're nearly frozen into place. We get stuck, so we may try to force our bodies into what we think are the correct positions. Thinking your way to a solution won't work; you need to feel your way there. You need to be able to observe yourself and feel your reactions. Don't think your body, feel your body. Observation is the key to change. You cannot fix something that you don't feel. This program is designed to help you feel your body again and allow it to adjust itself, not force it into another position. Observation is the key, and you can do that wherever you are.

Second, get as comfortable as you can and eliminate as many distractions as possible. In an ideal world, when starting this program, you would be wearing comfortable clothing and you would be in a quiet room. But we are living in the real world, so you may be reading this in a busy airport or at a convention center where quiet and comfort may not be possible. No matter. It will work in any context, but if there is anything you can do to improve conditions, you should.

Next, read the chapter on breathing. I know that it's tempting to skip over something that seems like second nature.

Please don't. Breathing is essential, and most of us don't realize the bad breathing habits we've developed. We hold our breath, take shallow breaths, and don't exhale fully. Holding your breath requires work, adding additional stress to your already taxed body. You must stop holding your breath in order to get relief. It's the foundation of my program.

Now, select a body part that you would like to work on. Turn to the chapter on that body part and choose the kind of movement that fits your circumstance. Note that within each chapter there are movements for standing, sitting, and lying down. If you are confined to a narrow airplane seat, you'll naturally use a seated move or ball placement. Be sure to select a body part that is conducive to resting on the ball; that is to say, if your back is in agony, you may want to choose another area. You may be better off starting with your elbow or your foot. You'll see as you use the program that your body is capable of creating amazing chain reactions—that it is possible to "reconnect" to your nervous system—and that your back can benefit from treatment applied elsewhere.

After you have placed the ball under part of your body, breathe, and let the weight of your body sink into the ball. You are following what I call Your Body Formula: Weight plus Breathing equals Release of Tension.

Your Body Formula
Weight + Breathing = Release of Tension

Focus on releasing your weight, on letting go. For many people, this is very difficult. Most familiar exercises and therapies involve forcing the body into a pose or a position, even if it feels painful or uncomfortable. No pain, no gain. My motto is the opposite: No pain, all gain. Think about release and about giving in, not about working and achieving results. All you have to do is stop holding your breath, let your weight go, give in to gravity, and observe your body's reactions.

You will note that throughout the exercises I ask you to take stock of what is happening in your body. This self-evaluation is an important part of the method. As I have tried to emphasize, you need to be able to feel your body. If you can feel it, then your body will be able to start adjusting it. Once your body realizes it's been holding itself, it knows how to release. Your body will begin to realign itself naturally.

You will notice that not all of the movements in the book require the ball. Throughout the book there are several of what I call Whole Body Moves. Normally the ball is used to let you feel your own weight and release the tension. But the Whole Body Moves do the same thing without the ball: They use gravity with the weight of your body to create a stretch throughout all your muscles and joints with one movement.

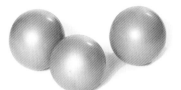

CHAPTER TWO

The Portable Prevention Prescription

D o these five moves every day, no matter where you are. They are marked throughout the book as Must-Do Moves. These Whole Body Moves do not require the ball, so you can do them anytime, anywhere. The focus should not be on exercise. Although it would be easy to mistake this sequence for an exercise routine, the focus should be on finding the target areas of your body to make sure you are truly moving them. One of the biggest mistakes people make in performing exercises is that they believe they are moving target areas, when, in fact, most of the time they are not, but are rather overusing the stressed muscles and underusing others. The result is chronic stiffness and little increase in flexibility and energy. Always remember Your Body Formula. You must feel your weight, and you must breathe in order to get benefits.

1 **Head and Neck Turns** (page 150): Target only your neck. Do not initiate the movement in your ribs, waist, or even shoulders. Your neck should rotate on your spine like a weather vane. The other parts may respond, but should not interrupt or prevent the movement.

2 **Raising Your Hands** (page 198): Focus on making your hands connect with your back. Don't let your shoulders inhibit the movement, but do let them move with your hands.

3 **Standing Body Hang Over** (page 108): This move is all about your hip joints and increasing their flexibility. Do not hang over at your waist; let the movement come from your hip joint. (If the situation doesn't allow the Standing Body Hang Over, try the Seated Body Hang Over on page 118.)

4 **Knee Bend for Back Relief** (page 120): This is to make you aware of your leg muscles and to make them more flexible so they can support your whole body.

5 **Standing Rib Stretch and Arch** (page 256): Pay attention to your middle back, entire ribcage, and releasing your diaphragm. This is to help you breathe easier and release the weight off your lower back.

Combine these moves and you can make this a routine to do every time you go on the ball or after breathing.

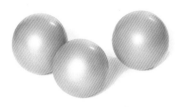

CHAPTER THREE

How to Breathe

I know it must be tempting to skip over a chapter on breathing. Please don't. Breathing is essential to the success of my program. Without it, the ball work is much less effective.

You might be thinking that you already know how to breathe; after all, you are alive, so you must be breathing. But how are you? Take a moment to notice how you breathe. Most of us hold our breath for much of the day. When we are not holding our breath, we tend to take in shallow breaths, and then do not exhale fully. The key to improving your breathing is exhalation. If you are able to empty your lungs fully, then you are able to refill them with fresh air. Think of a glass of water. If you never empty it, you can never refill it with new water. The more you learn to exhale, the stronger your diaphragm will become, and the stronger it becomes, the more effortlessly it will be able to draw breath in.

Breathing can (and should!) be done anywhere—sitting, standing, lying down; in your hotel room after a rough day, on a crowded plane, in the airport, while waiting in line, and so on. You don't need to clear time in your schedule to do it. One minute of the "S" Sound (page 53) is better than none and will offer you immediate benefits. It will begin to ease your muscle tension, will give you more energy, help you sleep, and calm you down in the midst of a stressful environment.

It may seem daunting to have to learn how to breathe. I have one observation and one bit of advice that I hope will help you. First the observation: It is impossible to hold your breath when you are on a ball and really letting it absorb your weight. If you are having trouble learning how to breathe, try doing it while resting on the ball. The advice: Try all of the breathing exercises in the book, then pick your favorite, and master just that one. You are better off mastering one exercise than dabbling with many.

Exercise One

- ## The "S" Sound
- ## relieves anxiety, muscle tension, and fatigue

1 Make an "S" sound as you exhale. It should sound like the hissing of a snake or a radiator letting out steam. Make the sound throughout the exhalation and make the exhalation as long as possible.

Notice how you make the sound. Do you find that you stiffen the muscles of your neck and shoulders? Or your jaw? Realize that this extra effort is unnecessary. On your next exhale focus on where the "S" sound really comes from.

2 What happens in between the sounds is what improves breathing. What do you notice? Give yourself a few breaths to observe. Then make the "S" sound again. Do you notice what part of your body helps you sustain the sound? Your diaphragm, the muscle that stretches beneath your ribcage like a drum, is what moves the air in and

out of your body. When you make the "S" sound, you tone your diaphragm, which enables you to pull more oxygen in and release more of it as well. It prevents you from breathing from your upper chest, which is the way most of us breathe, especially when we are rushing or under stress.

Notice if you have any reactions after you make the "S" sound. Are you yawning or sighing? Do you feel that you need to stretch your muscles as they begin to receive more oxygen? Are your eyes tearing? Is your nose running? Those are some of the most common effects of the "S" sound. Give yourself time to experience your body's reactions. And don't worry if you don't notice a difference right away. Continue to observe your body's response. Do you notice any muscles involved with your breathing?

If you don't get any reactions, that is fine, too. Notice, though, that nothing happened and just observe your regular breathing for a few extra breaths. Then make the sound again.

You don't have to make yourself breathe. Think "let it happen" not "force it deeper." It's your observation that creates change.

3 Make "S" sounds for 5, 10, 15, or even 20 minutes if you have the time. The longer you do it, the more results you will get. Your response to breathing is what relieves the muscle tension and stress. Give yourself that direction no matter how short a time you have. People want to fix themselves when they feel bad, but you have to allow your body to respond. *Do less, feel more.*

Exercise Two

- **The "F" Sound**
- **relieves anxiety, muscle tension, and fatigue**

Follow the instructions for the "S" sound, but instead of saying "ssssss," say "ffffffff." The beauty of the "F" sound is that it is more discreet (most people won't notice you are doing it if you choose to do it in public) but still requires your diaphragm to work. As with the "S" sound, take note of your body's reactions after each exhalation.

Exercise Three

- **Open Mouth Breathing**
- **relieves tight facial muscles, neck and shoulder tension, and headaches; soothes symptoms of TMJ; relaxes eye muscles for a rested appearance**

1 Hold your open hand a few inches from your mouth. Open your mouth and feel the weight of your jaw. Exhale for as long as you can, making a "haaaa" sound as though

you were trying to fog up a cold window. Right before the end of your exhalation, stop and gently close your mouth.

Note: You can use a fist instead of an open hand in front of your mouth. Putting your hand or fist in front of your mouth has two benefits: It enables you to feel the breath as you exhale, and it disguises what you are doing so that you don't have to feel uncomfortable about doing it in public.

2 Notice your response. Remember that observation is the key to change. Is your jaw stiff? Do this in front of a mirror if you have jaw tension. You may feel that your mouth is open, but it may not be. Your goal is to let it hang with the weight of gravity, not to force it open with your already overworked muscles.

3 Repeat for 5 minutes, or longer if you have time. Bring your hand up to your mouth and exhale, making a "haaaa" sound. Sustain the sound for the entire exhalation. Remember, do not force the breath out, just let it happen. (Don't think of it as an "exercise.") Notice any changes in your breathing. Connect the feeling of the jaw to your neck and shoulders.

Exercise Four

- **Exhaling through a Straw**
- **restores energy; improves muscle tone and posture; enhances flexibility; relieves stress**

1 Put a straw up to your mouth and exhale through it. Do not blow through the straw; simply allow the breath out naturally. Note that any kind of straw will do, from the smallest cocktail straw on up. The smaller the straw, the more gradually your diaphragm will contract.

2 Put the straw down and notice your reactions. You may have any number of reactions; see page 55 for the most likely reactions people have.

3 Inhale naturally, and then bring the straw back to your mouth and repeat. Do this for 5 to 10 minutes or more if you have the time.

Exercise Five

- **Tapping the Shoulder**
- **restores energy; relieves neck and shoulder tension; improves posture**

Tapping is an excellent way to start your day. When muscles become tight, the blood vessels near your skin constrict due to a lack of oxygen. Your muscles may feel achy, and they become more susceptible to injury. By tapping your body, you draw oxygen to the surface of the muscles. The feeling is restored, and the muscles are able to expand, which helps draw even more oxygen in.

1 Choose which side of your upper body you want to start with. If you have a tighter side, start with that one.

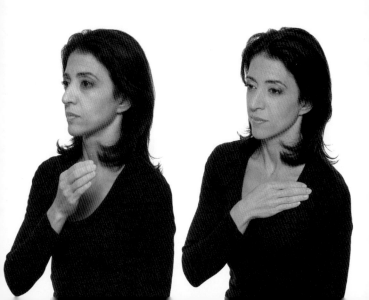

2 Cup your hand and tap in a circular motion the area above your breast and below your clavicle. Do this for a period of 15 seconds or so, then put your hand down, and pay attention to that part of your body. Has your breathing changed? Do the muscles that you tapped feel any different?

3 Repeat. Tap for another 15 seconds or so and notice your body's reaction. Do this for 2 to 3 minutes.

4 Move your hand up over the clavicle so that you are tapping from the hollow space just above the clavicle, over the top of

the shoulder, and onto your upper back. Support your elbow if you need to, and be sure not to stiffen your other shoulder while

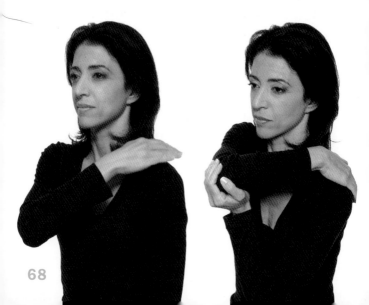

you tap. Tap for 15 seconds or so. Stop and notice your body's reaction. Do this for 2 to 3 minutes.

5 Move your hand underneath your armpit and tap up and down the side of your ribcage for 15 seconds or so. Stop and notice your body's reaction. Do this for 2 to 3 minutes.

6 Now, switch to the other side of your body and repeat the tapping in each area: front chest, upper shoulder, and ribcage. Make sure you take time to stop and notice your body's reaction. Tap on each area for

2 to 3 minutes. What do you notice? Do you feel the effects of breathing in that area of your body?

Note: You can do any part of this tapping exercise at any time you like. If you only have 2 minutes, just choose one part of your shoulder or ribcage and tap there for the 2 minutes. You will still feel relief. You can take all of these exercises à la carte as long as you follow the correct pacing and give yourself response time.

Exercise Six

- **Tapping the Breastbone**
- **restores energy; relieves stress; improves posture**

1 Relax your wrists, cup your fingers, and gently tap up and down the roughly six-inch span of your breastbone. (If you are sore or you experience discomfort, discontinue.)

2 Stop and notice your reactions. Has your breathing improved? Can you feel your breath in an unfamiliar area of your body, like your back? Do you have a clearer sense

of how you are sitting? Do you feel that you want to move? When muscles receive additional oxygen, they want to use it. Do not worry if you don't feel a strong reaction.

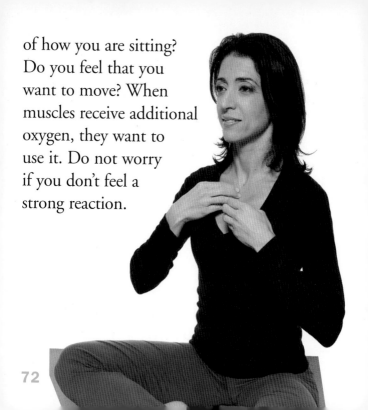

Let the breath flow through you, and other parts of your body will benefit.

3 Repeat the tapping, pausing to observe now and then, for 2 to 3 minutes.

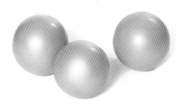

PART TWO

On the Ball

CHAPTER FOUR

Back

One of the common misconceptions about lower back pain is that the back muscles are weak and you need to strengthen both them and the muscles of the abdomen in order to create a "core" of support for your body. People think that the more you hold your body in perfect alignment, the more you will ease pain. In fact, holding and tightening and forcing your muscles into unnatural positions can greatly increase pain. Our bodies are not meant to be held tightly in a certain "aligned" position. Many of us are stuck in one position that we're unable to break out of, but our bodies are designed to move freely. Restoring the flexible connection of one part to the next is what gives you balance and frees you from pain.

The goal of the back section is to loosen your leg joints. When your leg joints are flexible, the muscles of the legs can support your lower back. Your weight is carried by your legs, not your lower back. Back on the Ball will make your breathing easier, and your diaphragm stronger. Your back will relax; your abdominal muscles will flatten; your waistline will narrow as your lower spine stretches out, and your legs will begin to support you instead of making your back do so much work.

Exercise One

- **Back on the Ball Lying Down**
- **relieves lower back ache; prevents muscle stiffness; promotes relaxation**

During this exercise, you may notice some small movements in your body as you rest on the ball. Most people do. Do not block the movements by clenching your muscles to try to stabilize yourself. These small movements mean that your body's natural realignment system is beginning to work. Your body is trying to find its balance. If the movements are becoming too big, and you feel like you will fall off the ball, it means that you are holding your breath and have lost the sense of your weight sinking into the ball. Make the "S" sound (page 53) and feel the weight of your body being absorbed by the ball. If you can't, come off the ball and start again.

1 To begin, lie on the floor and make the "S" sound (page 53). Notice any response your body might have to the "S" sound.

Let gravity take over. Be aware if you are holding parts of your body stiffly off the floor.

You can't move what you can't feel. You have to be able to feel in order to move.

2 Bend your knees and rest your feet flat on the floor. Notice how your legs affect your lower back. Take the ball, roll your pelvis to the side, and place the ball under the middle of the back of your pelvis. Roll up onto the ball. Note that the lower down on the back of your pelvis that you

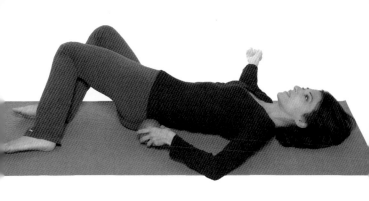

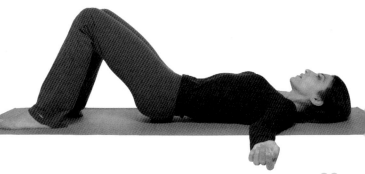

place the ball, the easier time you'll have releasing your weight into the ball. Feel the weight of your pelvis. Let your pelvis sink into the ball. How does your body react when you allow this part of it to rest on the ball? Take a moment to observe your body. Allow it to make adjustments. How do you know if you are doing it correctly? You'll find that when you truly allow a part of your body to rest on the ball, you cannot "stop" or "hold" your breath.

3 Make the "S" sound as you rest on the ball. Stay with this ball placement for 2 to 3 minutes.

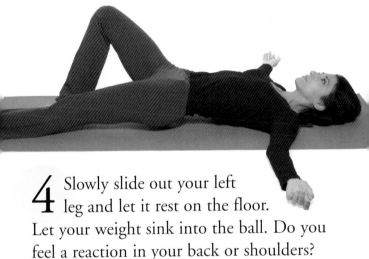

4 Slowly slide out your left
leg and let it rest on the floor.
Let your weight sink into the ball. Do you
feel a reaction in your back or shoulders?

5 Slowly flex your left ankle without
locking your knee joint. Notice that
your hamstring is beginning to stretch. After

Tension has a range. Just as you adjust the speed of your car to the conditions of the road, so should you adjust your muscle tension to your needs. You don't need big tension for small movements. Adjust your levels of effort to ensure that muscles do not get fatigued and that they stay flexible. Be creative with how you engage.

about 15 seconds, let your ankle release. Bend your left leg again so that the foot is resting flat on the floor. Note that it is essential that you do not lock your knee. If you lock your knee you will lock your hip

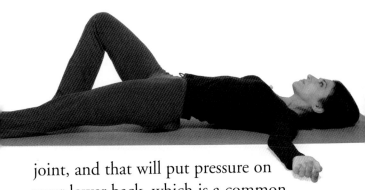

joint, and that will put pressure on
your lower back, which is a common
cause of lower back pain and stiff legs.

6 Repeat on your right side: Slide your
right leg out and feel the weight of the
leg rest on the floor. Do you notice any
connection to the lower back, or your other
leg as you move? Slowly flex your right

ankle. Feel how you flex it. Do you stop breathing? Make the "S" sound. After 15 seconds or so of flexing, release your ankle. Do you feel a change anywhere in your body?

7 Bend your left leg back up and let your pelvis adjust. Make the "S" sound. Slowly bring both knees up to your chest

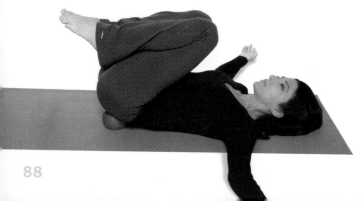

and lengthen your lower back. Allow your whole body to absorb the weight of your legs. Do not resist by stiffening your neck and shoulders and holding your breath. Notice that one movement affects your whole body. Rest in this position for 2 to 3 minutes. (If placement of the ball is painful, moving it slightly to another spot can make a huge difference, or try Calves on the Stool Lying Down on page 92.)

8 Bring your feet down one at a time. Roll your pelvis to the side and quickly take the ball away. It's important to remove the ball quickly so that you don't have time to

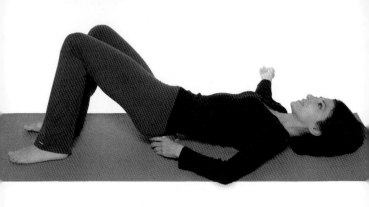

tense your muscles as you lower yourself
back to the floor. Slide both legs out and feel
your pelvis sink into the floor. How have
you changed? Observe your body's changes.
You don't have to do anything, just notice.

9 Repeat these movements 3 times. After the third time, leave the ball under your pelvis, and slide your legs straight out. Allow yourself to rest like this for as long as you can feel the benefits, 2 to 3 minutes.

It's better to do a thousand "wrong" movements every day than it is to have one way of holding yourself that you never move out of.

Exercise Two

- **Calves on the Stool Lying Down**
- **relieves sciatic problems, and hip and knee problems**

This is an incredibly relaxing, restorative exercise—perfect to do after a long travel day. Most hotel rooms have a coffee table or an ottoman that you can use to rest your calves on. The average height that's right for most people is about 15 inches. Do not do this exercise if you find that your feet are higher than your knees. Ideally, your calves should be parallel to the floor.

1 Lie on the floor and rest your calves on the coffee table, ottoman, or whatever you are using. Make sure that your feet are not higher than your knees and that your whole lower leg is being supported by the table. Your pelvis is now positioned so that your whole lower spine can release into the floor.

2 Make the "S" sound. As you exhale notice that your breathing is working to release tight muscles, which in turn allows gravity to help you sink into the floor.

If you are holding your muscles, you are holding your breath.

3 Take the ball in hand, roll your hip to one side, and place the ball under the middle of your pelvis. Rest and make the "S" sound. Let your pelvis sink into the ball.

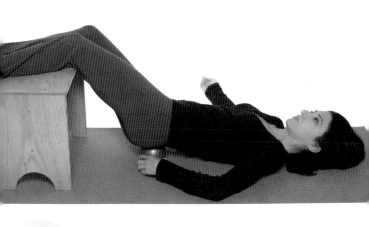

4 Allow your feet to come forward to the front of the coffee table. Let your thighs open up. Do not force your legs apart with your knees; instead, feel the weight of both thighs and see if you can

sense the connection to your hip joints and your lower back. Your hip joint is the foundation of movement for your whole body. If you start to feel there is too much pull in this joint, simply close your legs back to parallel and slide your calves back on the coffee table. If your knees hurt it means there isn't enough give in your hip joint yet. Return your legs to parallel and let them rest on the table. After a few moments of making the "S" sound in this position, try again and see if your joints are more willing to give in to the weight of your leg. Remember, don't force it. Remain with your

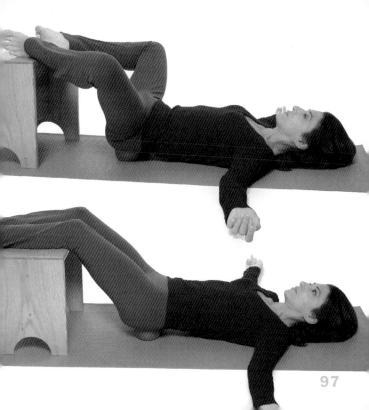

thighs opened up for as long as is comfortable, or 1 to 2 minutes.

5 Return your legs to parallel resting on the coffee table, roll your hip to one side, and quickly take the ball away. Let your weight sink into the floor. Make the "S" sound and notice any changes in your body.

Remember Your Body Formula: Weight + Breathing = Release of Tension. You must not hold your breath, so your muscles can relax and your body can self-adjust.

Exercise Three

- **Back on the Ball Seated**
- **promotes flexibility in the spine; relieves neck and shoulder tension; relieves back pain and stiffness**

This is ideal for travelers or those of us who find ourselves desk-bound for long stretches of time. Use the ball on a train, in a plane, or at your desk—anytime you find yourself in a high-backed seat.

1 While sitting, lean your body forward, take the ball up over your shoulder, and

drop it behind your back. Ideally it will land somewhere between your shoulder blades, but the exact location is not important. Then sit back and rest the weight of your body against it. Do not feel you have to push or attack the ball. The weight of your back will have enough effect. Adjust the ball if necessary.

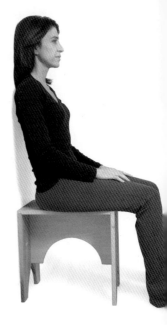

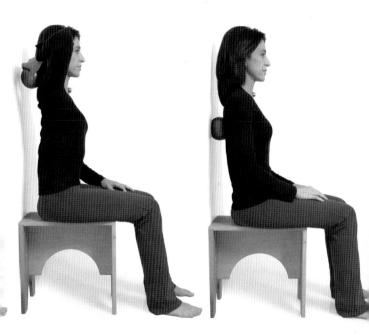

2 Do your favorite breathing exercise as you sink into the ball.

3 After 2 to 3 minutes lean forward a little and let the ball slide down your back a little farther. Give in to the ball for another 2 to 3 minutes. Observe your breathing.

4 Continue to repeat this sequence of leaning forward, letting the ball slide down, resting on it, and breathing until the ball has reached its lowest point on your back. At each point, remember Your Body Formula and notice any changes in your muscles.

If you notice any stiffening anywhere, give in to those areas. Notice if you are resisting and let your whole body respond to your breathing and your releasing into the ball. Any adjustments you notice may seem very subtle, but

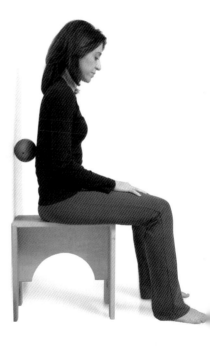

sometimes the smallest changes can be the most effective. It's all about relating one part of the body to the next.

5   At each stopping point of the ball's journey down your spine, consider adding a small movement of your head: Let your head rest back against the seat. Slowly turn your head to the right as far as your head will turn using just its own weight to turn it. Remember there is no such thing as an isolation exercise. Let the weight of your head turning move you to a new part on the ball. Don't force it. Let it rest there for 1 minute. Feel the connection between your

head and the muscles resting on the ball. Now turn your head to the left and feel the weight of it on that side.

6 When your head returns to the center, let its weight move it forward. As your head gently bends forward, allow

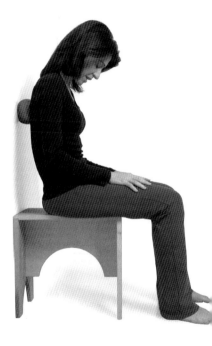

your back to sink deeper into the ball. When you pick your head back up, rest it against the seat. These small head movements help to slim waistlines, prevent the rounding of shoulders, and release lower back tension. Enjoy the breathing.

Remember to exhale.

7 Now take the ball away from your back and rest against the chair. Do you feel different parts of your body touching the chair now? Is your breathing different? Feel free to lift your hands up toward the ceiling.

Feel the connection between your arms and the muscles you were just resting on the ball. This will reaffirm that your body has a better range of movement than it did when you first sat down, and it also increases circulation throughout your entire body.

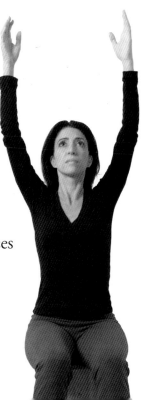

- **Standing Body Hang Over (Whole Body Move)**
- **relieves tight back muscles; stretches hamstrings; promotes flexibility; reshapes entire body**

The Standing Body Hang Over loosens leg joints, stretches hamstrings, prevents backaches, and energizes you. It is ideal for relieving lower back pain. And if you do it right, it will work every part of your body from the back of your heels to the back of your head. I do it all the time, no matter where I am. Remember Your Body Formula: Weight plus Breathing equals Release of Tension. There is no ball to sink into in this exercise; use the weight of your head and gradually your whole body as you come forward. Your goal is to let your leg joints bend. Do not push yourself aggressively or force yourself into a position. Just let gravity do the work, and your leg joints will follow.

1 Stand with your feet a little wider than hip distance apart. The closer together your legs are, the more difficult it is for you to bend at the hip joints.

2 Roll your head and body toward your toes, letting your arms hang. Give in to gravity. Let it pull your head, then your shoulders, ribcage, and ultimately your hip joints toward the floor. Your body will always bend at the joints, which it should, as long as you are giving in to gravity. This is one of the tighter areas of the body, so be patient with your body and give it time.

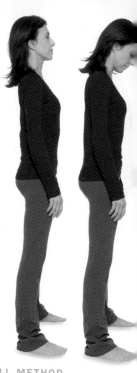

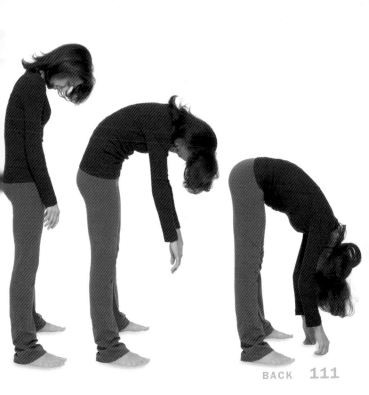

3 Bring your pelvis forward so that your hips are over your ankles. You can use a mirror to gauge how your hip joint bends if you need to. If your hips are behind your heels, your back is bearing most of the strain, and you are not stretching your hamstrings. If you have very tight hamstrings and you feel a powerful stretch, realize that your muscles are still resisting. You will need to work gradually to release them. Stay hung over for less time. Put your hands in front of you for support if your weight pulls you off balance. It is not important to be as flexible as the photos.

While you hang over, pay attention to your knees. In order to prevent yourself from locking your knees, bend them slightly when you are hanging over, then straighten them again. When you straighten them do not push the knee back behind the ankle, but rather straighten by lifting up the thigh muscle. If you feel that your knees are pronating, or turning inward, see page 120 (Knee Bend) for proper leg alignment.

4 Stay hung over as long as you feel the benefit. Know the difference between muscles releasing and muscles resisting. When a muscle is releasing, you sense

adjustments throughout your body; you can breathe; and you feel more stable. When a muscle is resisting, you feel uncomfortable; you can't breathe; and you feel like you are getting stiffer. If you feel stiff, come to standing and adjust yourself. If you feel a release, stay hung over for 1 to 2 minutes.

Your body talks to you in simple terms: with pleasure and pain. The ball is there to enable you to feel your body again. Once you can feel, you can make choices.

5 To come up, feel the weight of your feet going down into the floor. This will stabilize you as you come up to standing. Let your pelvis rotate up over your hip bones. I tell my students to imagine the pelvis rotating up around a rod that is going through the side of your hip and out the other, not unlike a rotisserie chicken.

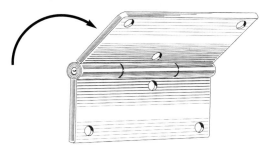

Variation One: Raised Heels

1 When you are in the Hang Over, you may lean forward onto your hands, palms flattened, and feel your heels come off the floor slightly. Your weight should be spread equally between your hands and your feet.

2 Raise your heels off the floor, stretching

into the balls of the feet. Move up and down 4 or 5 times.

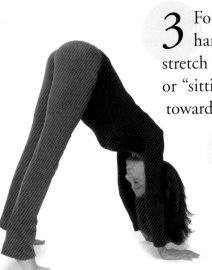

3 For an additional hamstring stretch, stretch your sit bones, or "sitting bones," up toward the ceiling.

4 With your sit bones raised, gently push into the left hip, then gently push into the right hip so your hips are moving side to side. Do this gently 3 or 4 times.

5 Walk your hands back to your feet until your feet are flat on the floor and come back up from the lower half of your pelvis.

Variation Two: Seated Body Hang Over

Try this movement when you don't have the space to do a Standing Body Hang Over.

1 Sit in a chair or cross-legged on the floor.

2 Roll your body forward over your legs. Start with the top of your head and neck and let them bend forward. When your torso is hanging over your legs, notice if you are holding your breath.

3 Sit up and your body realign itself. Let your body respond to feeling its weight and to your deeper breathing.

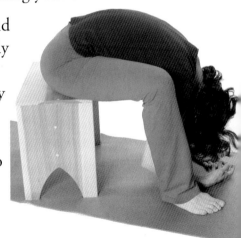

Exercise Five

- **Knee Bend for Back Relief (Whole Body Move)**
- **promotes proper leg alignment; relieves lower back pain and tired, stiff legs; changes the shape of your legs and body**

Most of us keep our knees locked when we are standing. This reinforces stiffness and causes weakness in the back and legs. The tighter your legs are, the more likely your back will hurt. Your legs have to be able to move in order to be supportive. This exercise helps make them supple.

One of my students once told me one of the most valuable lessons she learned in my class: There were so many times of the day, such as waiting in line, where she would normally just stand and be frustrated. After learning this move, she had something beneficial to do. By the time she would get to the checkout counter she would feel better than ever. This is an exercise you can do whenever you have a minute to spare.

1 Stand the way you normally do when waiting in line for a bus or at the store.

2 Leave your feet where they are, and slowly bend your knees, letting your ankles bend as well. Do not take any part of your feet off the floor.

3 Take a moment to notice where your knees are in relation to your toes. Are they pointing toward each other with your feet pointing away from each other? (This is common.) Your knees should be over your middle toes. If they are not, then the weight

of your body is being absorbed by your knees and lower back. Your feet are the giant shock absorbers of your body. So if your knee is not over your foot, your foot is not able to do its job, and the stress that it should be diffusing is heading right up your body to any number of places, such as your knees and back.

Remember to breathe.

4 Using your whole leg, begin to move your knees apart. You should feel that your inner thigh muscles and the muscles around the hip joints at the tops of your legs

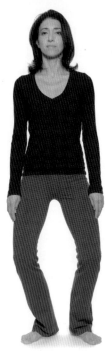

are involved in moving the knees. Stop when you feel that if you dropped a plumb line from the tip of your knee, it would hit your middle toe. You will notice when your knees are aligned properly that the outsides of your feet are absorbing more of your weight. There should be much less pressure on your big toes, and you may notice more of an arch in your feet.

5 After you have aligned your knees over your middle toes, slowly start to push against the floor to straighten your legs and lift your body up. When you notice that your feet want to start rolling in and your knees start to cave in, you've gone too far. Bend your knees, align them, and then straighten up again a few times. Every time you start to revert to your old habit, stop and practice this new way of standing and alignment.

Note that no two bodies do this the same way. You have to be aware of how you move so you can give your body new choices of movement. Then try to lift up using different muscles than you usually do. For example, feel your feet firmly against the floor; lift your quads; and use your whole body to straighten your legs. This movement connects your legs to your pelvis, so you may notice muscles at the bottom of your pelvis or top of the legs engaging that you have never felt before. Try to use this revised lift every time you bend your knees.

This is one movement in particular in which you may notice unfamiliar feelings in your body. That is good, but forcing movement or feeling pain is not good, so listen to your body. You may be introducing yourself to muscles or body parts you didn't know you had. Once you discover these new parts, you can communicate better with your body when you do Miracle Ball moves or your favorite sports. Instead of using (and overusing) the same muscles you always do, you'll have more choices and different ways to support your body.

CHAPTER FIVE

Neck and Head

Most of us spend our days looking down. We are looking down at our children or hunching over our computers. We are poring over the map or digging down for our keys. Children, on the other hand, spend their days looking up. They are looking up to admire Mom, to catch a ball, or to see high into trees. Their ribcages are lifted off of their diaphragms; they have flexible wrists and hands; and they have waistlines. The lift in their bodies enables them to breathe effortlessly, which gives them energy and enhances muscle tone. We adults need to remember what it's like to look up. We need to stop hunching, rounding our upper backs forward, and sinking our chests in. Lifting will restore feeling in the head and neck, and create a sense of well being. Your back and lower body will feel better when you learn to look up again.

Exercise One

- **Head on the Ball Lying Down**
- **improves posture; relieves tension headaches; relieves neck and shoulder tension; helps relieve wrist and hand pain, too**

This ball placement is great for traveling. Have the ball in bed with you. Wake up and place it under your head. Release the jaw and start the day on the ball.

1 Lie down and place the ball under your head. Remember Your Body Formula (page 38) and place the ball where it can

fully support the weight of your head. Move it around until you find the best place. Allow your body to adjust, sink, and give in to the ball.

2 Rest there and make the "S" sound. Give in to the weight of your head. Sense if you feel reactions in any other parts of your body. Feel the connection between one part of the body and another.

3 Move your head slowly as though you were shaking your head "no" to someone in slow motion. Make your head initiate the movement, not your neck. Let your jaw and the front of your neck slacken. Drop the back of your ribcage between your shoulders toward the floor. Repeat 4 or 5 times.

Remember you initiate the movement from the part of your body that is resting on the ball.

4 Now, move your head slowly as though you were nodding "yes" to someone in slow motion. Do this 4 or 5 times.

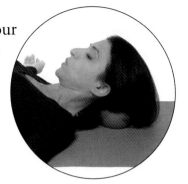

5 Take the ball away and rest your head on the floor. Notice if any parts of your body are resting differently on the floor than when you first lay down. Do you have a breathing reaction?

It's not about the movement.
It's about what effect the
movement has on your body.

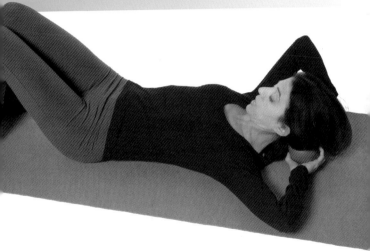

Exercise Two

- **Face on the Ball**
- **eases the pain of TMJ and tension around the eyes; improves posture**

1 Lie on your stomach and rest your forehead on the ball. Place your arms over your head with your elbows bent slightly so your shoulders can be at ease. Make sure you are not stiffening your neck

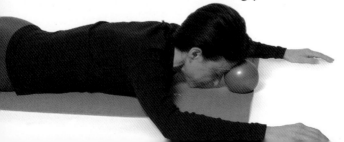

muscles. Let your neck bend as your head adjusts to the ball. Breathe.

2 Slowly turn your head to the left using its weight to guide you. When your head is turned as far as it can comfortably go, rest there for a minute. Feel free to adjust the position of the ball at any time for your comfort. Remember, you need to be able to feel the weight of your head sinking into it.

3 Slowly turn your head back to center and then turn it to the right side. Rest on the right for a minute. Do you feel a reaction in any other parts of your body?

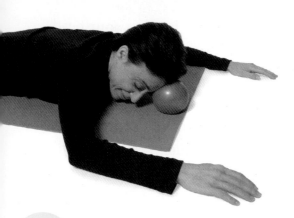

4 Move the ball and rest your chin on it. Slacken your neck and feel the back of your neck soften. Breathe. Stay here for a few minutes and notice what happens in other parts of your body.

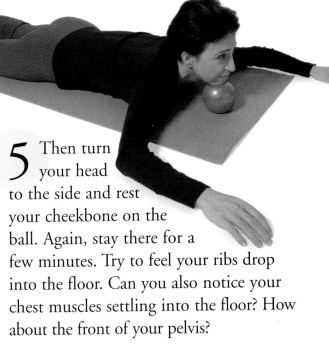

5 Then turn your head to the side and rest your cheekbone on the ball. Again, stay there for a few minutes. Try to feel your ribs drop into the floor. Can you also notice your chest muscles settling into the floor? How about the front of your pelvis?

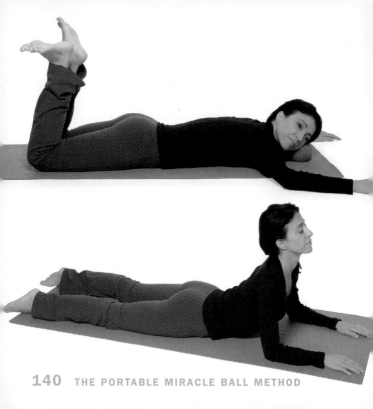

6 Bend your knees and rotate your ankles in circles. Let your weight sink into the floor. Do this for 1 to 2 minutes, then put your legs back on the floor.

7 Using your hands, push up and reach the top of your head toward the ceiling. Do not lift your spine like a plank. Place your elbows underneath your armpits, feel the sternum move forward, your head lift, and the weight of the pelvis dropping down. You should resemble a sphinx. Slowly turn your head right and left. If you like, you may push all the way up into straightened

arms, lengthening from your pubic bone through your forehead. Remember, for movement to be beneficial it shouldn't be forced. Experiment with different styles, ways of moving, and speed, and adjust your body with each movement.

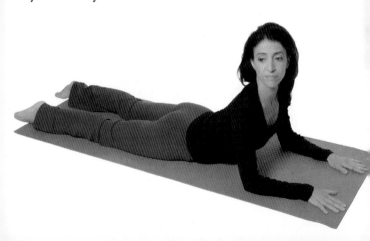

8 Uncurl your whole body until you are lying flat with your forehead or cheek on the floor. Breathe. Notice that you can feel the breath throughout your back.

9 Now roll onto your back and place the ball behind your head. Open your mouth gradually on an exhalation. Sustain a gentle "haaaa" sound.

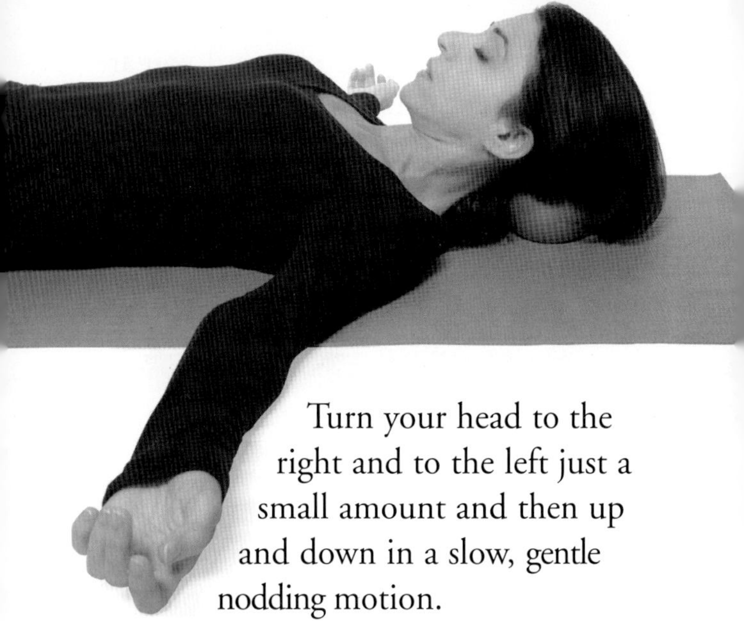

Turn your head to the
right and to the left just a
small amount and then up
and down in a slow, gentle
nodding motion.

10 Come to a sitting position. Open your mouth and let your jaw hang open. Breathe and notice any changes your body has made.

It's better to take more time doing one exercise and get real results than to rush through many different exercises. What you are looking for is the feeling of relief. True relief in one part of the body will have a positive "domino effect" throughout your whole body.

Exercise Three

- **Neck on the Ball Seated**
- relieves stiff neck muscles; relaxes upper back tension; promotes better breathing posture

1 Place the ball on top of your shoulder next to your neck and rest your head on the ball. Let the weight of your head sink into the ball. Then do Open Mouth Breathing for 2 to 3 minutes.

2 Repeat on the other side.

3 Move the ball to the back of your neck where the back of your head meets the top of your spine. (Note that you must be

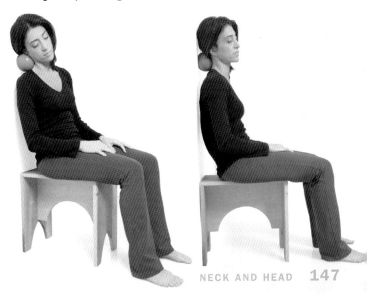

in a chair with a high back
in order to do this.) Let the
weight of your head and
whole body sink into the
ball. Breathe. Give in like this
for as long as you feel at ease.

4 Remove the
ball and let
your head sink
forward toward
your chest.
Let your neck
soften and

let your chin bend forward with the weight of the top of your head. Breathe. Stay like this for 2 to 3 minutes.

5 Repeat this sequence 3 or 4 times.

Pain is caused by holding your body in one position for too long. Allow your body to shift when you are on the ball.

- **Head and Neck Turns (Whole Body Move)**
- **lengthens neck muscles; reduces stress; improves posture and breathing**

You can do this exercise standing or sitting.

1 Start with the tighter side of your neck and turn your head as slowly as possible toward it. Go as far as you comfortably can and then return to center. Are you tightening your shoulders and stopping your breathing as you do it? Focus on breathing

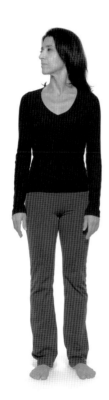

and not involving your shoulders in the movement. Many of us think we are moving our necks when in fact we simply pull the shoulder toward the face and twist at the waist. Keep your body at ease so that only your head is turning. Picture a weather vane whose base stays in place while the arrow moves gently with the wind.

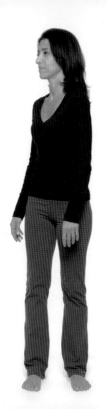
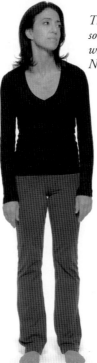

These photos illustrate some positions to avoid when doing Head and Neck Turns.

2 Repeat several times on that side. Can you allow your body to adjust? Do you notice any changes in your body? Let your body respond to them. Breathe.

3 Repeat the exercise on the other side.

4 Finally, let the weight of your head bend forward. Let your ribcage press into the chair if you are sitting, or round slightly if you are standing. Do you feel anything in your upper back? Finish by tilting your head backward and looking up.

CHAPTER SIX

Shoulders

When many people think of good posture, they throw their shoulders back, squeeze the blades together, and push their chests forward. This actually causes more stiffness in the body. Good posture should originate from your whole body, not just your shoulders. The shoulders should simply rest on top of the body, with the arms dangling free.

Stiff shoulders can make it difficult to breathe and may cause headaches, jaw pain, and back tension. Many ailments that appear to relate to the hands and wrists, like carpal tunnel syndrome, are actually more related to this very overworked area. If you have any ailment from the neck to the fingers for which you seek relief, do not overlook the shoulder exercises in this book. They may be just what you need to pinpoint your trouble spot.

Exercise One

- **Ball Between the Shoulder Blades Lying Down**
- **relieves upper back and neck stiffness; improves breathing and posture; restores energy; boosts flexibility**

1 Lie on the floor on your back. Bend your knees and rest your feet on the floor. Take a moment to notice how your shoulders rest on the floor. Is one shoulder higher than the other? Are you breathing? Is there a big gap between your shoulder blades? If parts

of your body are off the floor, recognize that your muscles are keeping them off the floor.

2 Make the "S" sound and give your body a moment to respond. Feel how your muscles take in the oxygen. Feel your weight sinking into the floor. Make the "S" sound again and notice your body's response. Do this for 3 to 5 minutes.

Exercise Two

- **Deep Shoulder Stretch**
- **improves rotation of the shoulder blade; takes pressure off the mid back; improves posture; creates flexibility in the spine**

1 Lie down on your back. Take the ball in one hand, roll your body to one side, and place the ball in between your shoulder blades. Higher up the back is easier than lower down the back. If you feel discomfort, try shimmying down on the ball so that it is higher on your back. The back of the

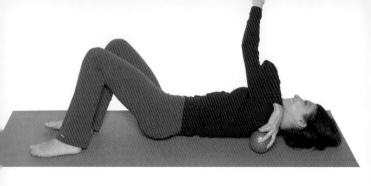

ribcage between the shoulder blades is usually
one of the tightest areas of the body. It's what
I think of as a hot spot. When you let yourself
breathe and allow your body to drape over the
ball, you'll start to feel how much tension you
hold in your body all day and how flexible
the areas of your upper back, shoulders, and

neck can be. You should begin to be able to distinguish the different parts of your upper body from the knot that they so often make. Rest this way as long as it is comfortable, 1 to 2 minutes for beginners.

2 Remove the ball and feel your weight sink into the floor. Are your shoulders resting differently? Is your breathing different? Do you notice any other effects?

3 Get back on the ball, placing it off center, toward the tighter shoulder. It should be resting between your shoulder blade and spine. Let your body drape over

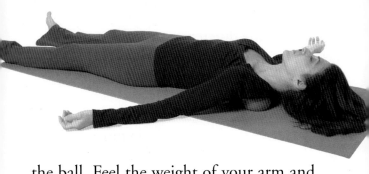

the ball. Feel the weight of your arm and hand. Make the "S" sound.

4 Reach your arm that is closest to the ball toward the ceiling. Do not stiffen the elbow. Notice the relationship of your back to the ball. Have you pulled some of

Travel is a real opportunity for Miracle Ball Method fans. There is usually lots of down time in which you can be using the ball or doing Whole Body Moves. Do your breathing.

your weight from the ball? Have you stopped breathing? If you bend your elbow and slightly soften your wrist, you will feel the weight of your shoulder and upper back rest more comfortably on the ball. Then reach through your hand again, lengthening but not stiffening your arm. Feel the connection to

your upper back muscles. Again, slightly bend
your elbow, feel the ball absorb your weight,
then reach through again. Repeat 3 times.

5 Let your arm drape across your chest
and rest. Let your head turn in the
direction of your arm. Feel your weight
press into the ball. Make the "S" sound.

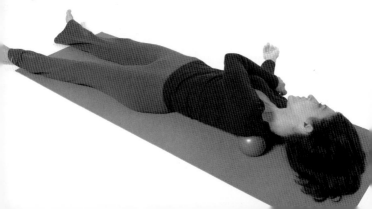

6 Circle
your hand up
over your head and notice
the movement in your upper back
and shoulder as you go. Note that you
cannot fully rotate your shoulder if the rest
of your body is stiff and you are holding
your breath. So feel the weight of your body
and breathe as you do this. Stop with your
arm over your head and rest there for a

moment. Then take your hand back to shoulder level and move your arm parallel to your body.

7 Take the ball away, let your weight sink into the floor, and notice if your shoulders are resting any differently on the floor. Has your breathing changed? It is important to take the time to notice any changes in your breathing and your body. Rest for 1 to 2 minutes.

8 Repeat on the other side of your body.

Exercise Three

- **Shoulder on the Ball, Seated and Standing**
- **improves flexibility of shoulders; improves breathing and posture**

This movement can be done standing or sitting. The instructions are written for sitting, but you can easily adjust them for standing.

1 First, take stock of your body. How are you breathing? Are you stiff anywhere? Do your open mouth breathing: Make the

"S" sound or choose your favorite breathing technique.

2 Take the ball and place it between your shoulder blades in the middle of your back. Press into the chair. Feel your head resting against the seat, and feel your weight sink into the ball and the chair. Breathe. Give your body time to rest in this position.

3 Let your head roll from right

to left, very slowly. Stop on one side and feel the connection between your back and your head. Slowly roll to the other side and do the same. Feel the weight and breathe.

4 Take your right hand and rest it on your left shoulder. Move your head to the left. Feel the weight and breathe. Slowly move your elbow slightly away

from your chest and toward the ceiling. Then lower it and see if your arm sinks a little closer to your chest. Move your arm down, then reach it up toward the ceiling without stiffening your elbow joint. Feel how your shoulder connects to your upper back.

5 Repeat with your left hand. If you can, spend 5 minutes with

this. If you have more time, try to do it for 15 minutes.

A Word about Chairs

Many of my students are concerned that once they start feeling better, they have to keep their alignment. They worry especially about chairs. They think that there is a specific alignment they should be holding that will prevent pain caused by hours spent confined in uncomfortable theater, airline, and car seats. This is not true. Actually, what causes pain is forcing your body into an alignment. This causes stiffness and makes you hold your breath. You are better off sinking into the chair and letting yourself breathe, even if it makes a curve in your back. Your body was designed to move into millions of different positions. It's not the positions that are causing your pain. It's the way you are holding yourself— your breath and your body—that causes pain. So rather than working to hold your alignment while at the theater or on a plane, work at *not holding your breath.*

CHAPTER SEVEN

Wrists and Hands

The flexibility of your wrists and hands depends upon the flexibility of your shoulders and upper back, and vice versa. It is important that as you do wrist and hand movements you remember not to stiffen your shoulders. I also suggest that, if you suffer from any condition of the hand, elbow, shoulder, or upper back, you try any of the ball placements in all of these chapters. You may think a problem relates to your fingers, but in fact, it might be originating closer to your spine.

I also point out to my students that people tend to keep their hands clenched for much of the day. I suggest to them, as I do to you, that when you do the Standing Body Hang Over (page 108), you concentrate on feeling the weight of your hands at the ends of your arms. This will stretch your back muscles greatly and boost your circulation.

Exercise One

- **Wrist on the Ball Lying Down**
- **eases shoulder tension and carpal tunnel syndrome; improves breathing; loosens muscles of mid back**

1 Lie on the floor and make the "S" sound. Bring your attention to your hands. Are they clenched even when the body is at rest? Notice what knuckle you are resting on. Realize that any part of your body that hurts is a reflection of your whole body. Notice not only your hands, but also your arms, your shoulders, your back. They

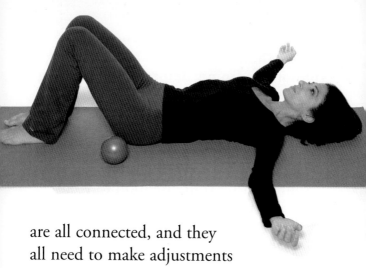

are all connected, and they
all need to make adjustments
in order for your hands to feel relief.
Make the "S" sound again and observe
your body's reactions.

2 Then, as slowly as you can, take the backs of your hands slightly up off the floor, just enough to sense their weight, then release them back to the floor. Notice if you feel more of a connection to any other parts of your body. Some people stiffen up many parts of their bodies when

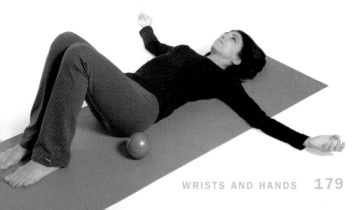

they raise their hands. Try lifting just your hands again while letting your shoulders and arms release their weight into the floor.

3 With your arm resting about a foot from the side of your body, drape your hand, palm facing down, over the ball. Your wrist should be the primary

point of contact. Stay like this and notice the changes in the rest of your arm and shoulder. Notice that when you brought your hand alongside your body and over the ball, there were changes in your upper back and shoulder area.

4 Slowly raise your knuckles up toward the ceiling and feel the weight of your wrist press into the ball. Release the weight again and allow your body to give in. Some body parts may make adjustments. Let them. Notice whether you are holding your breath. Remember that there are only two

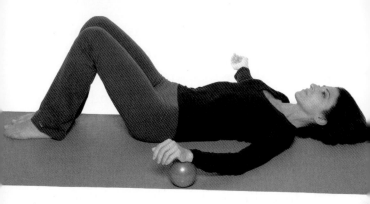

choices: You can either keep every body
part in place, or you can let your body parts
shift. Lift your wrist up and release down
giving time in between. Do this for 3 to 5
minutes, breathing, and notice any changes.

5 Lift your wrist and hand off the ball and move your arms to their original outstretched positions. Do you notice any changes? Breathe.

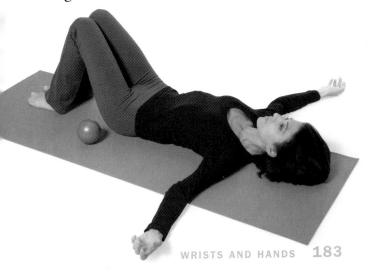

Exercise Two

- **Elbow on the Ball Lying Down**
- **restores motion to the shoulder joint; eases tension in upper back, shoulder, and arm**

1 Lie on your back. Bend your elbow so your palm is facing the ceiling and the joint is roughly at a 90-degree angle. Place the ball under your upper

arm between your elbow and shoulder.
Breathe and let your weight sink into the
ball. Has your shoulder shifted its position?
Remain like this for as long as you feel
comfortable and notice changes in your body,
ideally for at least 2 to 3 minutes.

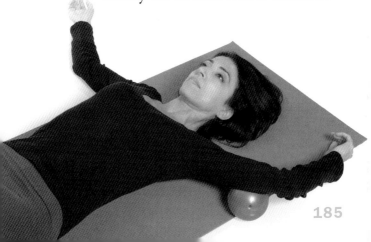

2 Remove the ball and stretch your arms out. Breathe and notice any changes.

3 Go on and off the ball 2 or 3 times on each side of your body.

Remember: Most of your reactions will happen as you let your body give in and you clench less. Feel that domino affect through your whole body.

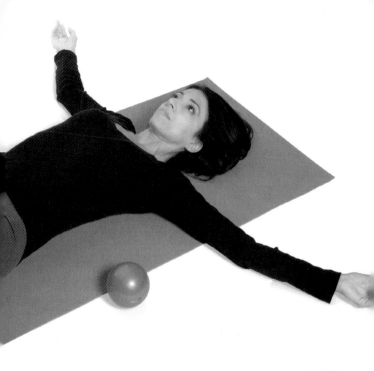

Exercise Three

- **Wrist on the Ball Seated**
- **eases shoulder tension and carpal tunnel syndrome; improves breathing; loosens muscles of mid back**

This is perfect for when you are at your desk or on an airplane with your tray table down.

1 Drape your wrist over the ball. Keep your arm and shoulder as loose as possible. The goal is to allow every body part to self-adjust.

2 Raise up your hand and press your wrist into the ball. Make sure your arm and shoulder are responsive as you do this. Take your hand off the ball and let it rest in your lap. Let your weight sink into your hand. Do you feel different? Breathe. Do several repetitions of the wrist lift, removing your hand

from the ball after each one to take stock of how your body feels.

3 Repeat with your other hand.

Variation One: As you rest your wrist on the ball, you can take your other hand up to your opposite shoulder and tap it, front and back, for about 15 seconds. (See page 65.) Notice how your shoulder eases up after you tap and your breathing becomes easier. Stiff, tight shoulders make breathing difficult and inhibit the motion of your arms and hands. Repeat on the other side.

Variation Two: Another thing you can do while you rest your wrist on the ball is to move one finger at a time slowly up toward the ceiling and then release it back down. Try to make each finger move separately (this will be easier with some fingers than others). Make sure that after you release each finger, you take stock of how your body feels. Are you letting your arm hang loosely?

Are you still breathing? Are you letting the weight of your fingers be absorbed by the ball?

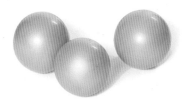

Exercise Four

- **Ball Under the Armpit**
- **eliminates round shoulder pose; keeps you limber in cramped spaces; improves breathing; prevents fatigue**

This exercise can be done seated or standing and is a great pose for tight seated conditions, such as commuter trains and airplanes. It is also excellent for use at the computer, as it keeps the shoulder and upper back from getting stiff.

1 Place the ball between your upper arm and the side of your rib cage. It should

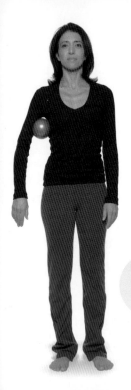

be a comfortable distance from your armpit. Breathe. If you have room, you can let your forearm hang free. If you are in a confined space, let your hand rest in your lap. Feel the weight of your arm sink into the ball. Is your shoulder dropping? Is your back less round?

2 Take the ball away. Do you feel the weight of your upper arm drawing your shoulder down?

Is there a difference between your two shoulders? Do you want to move your head to let your neck readjust?

3 Put the ball back. Try to go on and off the ball for 3 to 5 minutes.

4 Repeat on the other side of your body.

Variation One: You can only do this variation if your arm is hanging free. With the ball under your arm, gently rotate your upper arm where you are pressing against the ball so that your shoulder turns inward,

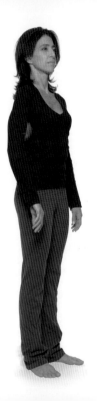

and then outward. Do this very, very slowly. Take the ball away and notice any changes. Breathe.

Variation Two: After removing the ball from under your arm, gently shrug your shoulder up toward the ceiling. Your arm should be draping from your shoulder, not shoving upward toward your rear. You will feel a connection to your back if you initiate this movement from your shoulder rather than your arm.

5 Finish by reaching both hands at the same time up toward the ceiling. Don't stiffen your arms. Reach with your hands and fingers and let your arms follow. Feel how your whole spine is lifted and how your head adjusts itself in relation to your whole torso lifting up instead of hunching forward.

- **Raising Your Hands (Whole Body Move)**
- **restores energy; improves posture and flexibility; trims waistline**

While sitting during your day, stop and raise your arms into the air. This lifts the ribcage off the diaphragm, allowing breath to come more easily. Without the breath, the upper back will remain stiff. You can do this exercise in a chair or standing.

1 Raise your hands up toward the ceiling, remembering that they connect directly

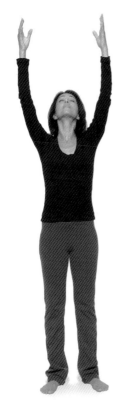

to your back. Do not stiffen your elbows and shoulders. You should feel a sense of your ribcage lifting up off your diaphragm. Tilt your head and look up if that helps you feel a stronger connection between your hands and your back. Remember that this is a Whole Body Move. You should allow a chain reaction to spread throughout your body. Let more parts of your body get involved. Breathe and let your body make adjustments if it wants to. Feel your spine lengthen.

2 Bring your arms down but do not feel that they need to pull your whole body back into its original hunched position.

3 Repeat 3 times or whenever you have the chance throughout your day.

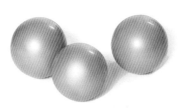

CHAPTER EIGHT

Hips, Legs, and Feet

The hip joint is the body's foundation of movement. Your hips, along with your legs and feet, are the shock absorption system of your body. If they do not remain limber and flexible, your back will end up absorbing all the stresses of your everyday movements. Many people with back pain don't realize that their problems stem more from their tight hip joints and hamstrings than from their backs.

By relieving tension in these parts of your body, you will relieve tension in many others as well, especially the lower back. The movements in this chapter are essential for travelers, whose legs and hips need to remain supple in order to support a body on the go.

Exercise One

- **Hamstring Release Lying Down**
- **relieves fatigue, stiffness, and tight hamstrings; boosts flexibility; relieves symptoms of sciatica**

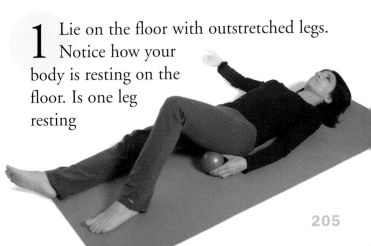

1 Lie on the floor with outstretched legs. Notice how your body is resting on the floor. Is one leg resting

differently than the other? Start with the leg that seems tighter.

2 Start at the top of your thigh. Bend your knee slightly and place the ball under the top of your thigh. Breathe and give your leg a chance to soften into the ball. You may notice that your leg begins to rotate outward. As you rest on the ball, notice if you feel other parts of your body responding, such as your hip, knee, ankle, or foot. Remember not to hold your breath.

3 After 2 to 3 minutes, push the ball down to the middle of your thigh between your hip joint and knee. Give it time to rest on the ball. Make the "S" sound and let your leg adjust, which it may do again by rotating outward. Rest 2 to 3 minutes.

4 Push the ball down so it is just above your knee. Rest there, breathing, and let your weight sink into the ball for 2 to 3 minutes. Again, you may notice the muscles of your hip joint lengthen, so allow your leg to rotate outward.

5 If you have time, you can continue pushing the ball down your leg. The next stop should be behind your calf, between your knee and ankle. Use your other foot to push the ball into place. If your leg feels wobbly, you are stiffening it. You must let the weight of your calf sink

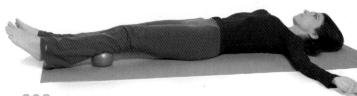

into the ball. Adjust the ball so that your knee loosens and your hip joint is able to rotate your leg outward. Many of my students feel that their knees are bent severely and pointing outward at a sharp angle in this position, but if you lift your head up and look, you'll find that the leg is actually pretty straight. Your knee is now lined up with your foot and hip. It only feels like a strong turnout because most people's knees are so pronated, or turned inward. If this exercise makes you realize that you are usually pronated, you will also benefit from the Knee Bends on page 120.

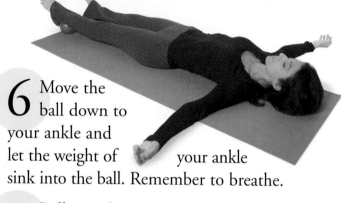

6 Move the ball down to your ankle and let the weight of your ankle sink into the ball. Remember to breathe.

7 Pull your knee out to the side and drop its weight to the outside of your ankle and rest on the ball there. Your knee should be as loose as possible. Do you feel this loosening your hip? Breathe and rest here a few minutes.

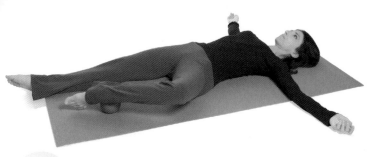

8 If you feel stable, you can very gently and slowly roll the ball under your out-turned ankle. Feel free to wiggle your toes and flex your foot. Finish by stretching your leg out to return your weight to the back of your ankle.

9 Repeat on the other side.

Exercise Two

- **Ball Between the Knees Lying on Side (Hip Release)**
- **relieves hip pain (especially good for pregnant women), low back ache, and general back tension; great for bed, to relieve stiffness in the legs**

This is great emergency relief for a sudden back spasm. If lying on your back or getting on the floor is difficult, do this in bed on your side. It will gradually relax the spasm by creating a better breathing reaction every time you take the ball away.

1 Lie on your side. Do not hunch forward. Soften your bottom shoulder and roll slightly back on your ribcage and the back of your head so that you are not pulling forward with your neck and jaw. Breathe. Feel your weight sink into the floor.

2 Bend your knees so they are approximately at a 90-degree angle. Take the ball, slowly raise your top leg, and place the ball between your knees. Rest there, letting your weight sink into the ball. If you are uncomfortable, try moving the ball higher than your knee, or lower, until

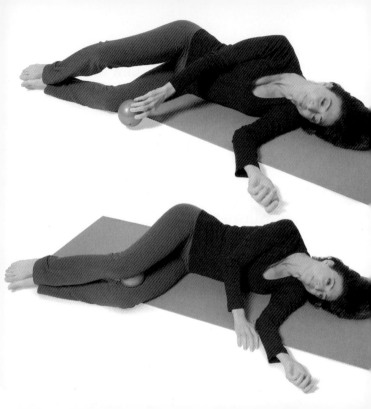

you feel comfortable. Breathe. Notice if you sink more into the ball. Do your hips or your lower back feel different?

3 Lift your top knee just enough to take the ball away. Gradually release the weight of your leg so that it is resting on your bottom one. Breathe. Give in to gravity.

4 Repeat 3 times, moving slowly and gradually each time. Are you able to release your leg more easily? Are you feeling a connection to your back? Can you feel your breath there?

Exercise Three

- **Instep on the Ball Lying Down**
- **relieves stiff, tired feet; helps realign the leg with the foot; creates flexibility throughout the leg and hip; supports lower back**

1 Lie on your stomach and place the ball on the front of one of your insteps (the top of your foot will be on ball). If you have a tighter side, start on that side. Breathe. Note that it is easier to feel breathing in the lower half of your body when you are on your stomach. Your other foot should be at ease.

2 Notice whether you are clenching the muscles of your buttocks. Release them. The goal is to let your thigh bone rest more easily in its socket by releasing the tight muscles that surround the joint. Many people joke that their bottoms are flabby and have no muscles at all. This is not true! In fact, if the muscles closest to the bone are clenched, the muscles at the surface remain unused and flabby. Our goal is to ease the stiffness closer to the joint so that you can have a more balanced tone.

3 Make the "S" sound and give in to the weight of your body. Spend 2 to 3 minutes doing this and notice the way your hips and thighs are resting on the floor as your instep drapes over the ball.

4 Gently stretch your foot out by reaching through your toes and then let your foot drape back over the ball. Do this 2 to 3 times, making sure that you release each time in between and that you are doing your breathing.

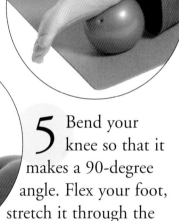

5 Bend your knee so that it makes a 90-degree angle. Flex your foot, stretch it through the ball of your foot and toes, and then make gentle circles with it. Breathe. Do this for several minutes.

Variation:

1 Try this variation if you feel very flexible: If you are working on your left foot, roll onto your right side; if you are working on your right foot, roll onto your left side. Use your foot to push the ball up to your hand. Bend your knee at a 90-degree angle. Use your hand to place the ball under your knee. Roll forward onto the ball. Breathe and rest here for 2

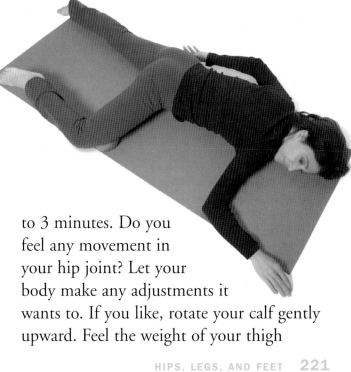

to 3 minutes. Do you
feel any movement in
your hip joint? Let your
body make any adjustments it
wants to. If you like, rotate your calf gently
upward. Feel the weight of your thigh

pressing into the ball. This heightens the rotation in your hip. Each time you release, notice your muscles. Are they looser? Are you letting your weight go into the ball? Are you breathing?

2 Take the ball away. Stretch out your legs. Compare sides. Breathe.

3 Repeat the whole exercise with your other foot.

Exercise Four

- **Hamstring Release Seated**
- **helps prevent leg cramps; boosts circulation in legs; keeps the hip joint flexible**

This exercise is great for planes, trains, and automobiles (but not for the driver!). Use any time when you are going to be seated for a long time.

1 Lean back into your chair and get comfortable. Lift your knee up and place the ball as high up the back of your

thigh as possible. Breathe and let your leg sink into the ball.

2 Move the ball a little lower down your thigh toward your knee. Let the leg rotate outward if it wants to. You must feel your weight and continue to breathe in order for the leg to release. If you have room, stretch your leg out a little bit

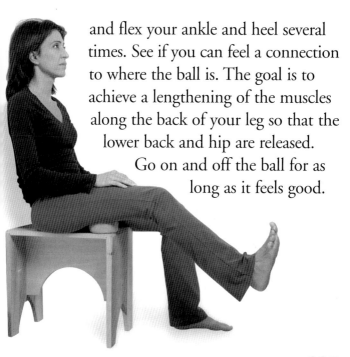

and flex your ankle and heel several times. See if you can feel a connection to where the ball is. The goal is to achieve a lengthening of the muscles along the back of your leg so that the lower back and hip are released. Go on and off the ball for as long as it feels good.

3 Remove the ball and see if your leg is sitting lower in the seat than the other one. Breathe and let your body make adjustments.

4 If you have room, move the ball farther down your leg and repeat step two.

5 Repeat with your other leg.

Exercise Five

- **Foot and Ankle on the Ball Seated**
- **makes the foot more flexible for optimal shock absorption; loosens the hip joint, which takes pressure off of lower back; identifies and tones lesser-used muscles in the hip and thigh**

Feet are incredibly stiff, and they mirror the stiffness in the back and hamstrings. This exercise helps you release your foot and causes a chain reaction that runs up your legs to your back.

1 Put the ball under the arch of your foot. Sit back into your seat. Resist the urge to immediately roll your foot around on the ball. Give yourself time to let your foot sink into the ball. Make the "S" sound. Notice the relationship between your foot, knee, and hip.

2 Let your foot sink into the ball. Soften your ankle and release any stiffness in your toes. When you do this, you will feel

that more of your foot is making contact with the ball, and you will notice that your foot can begin to move.

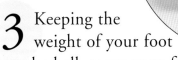

3 Keeping the weight of your foot on the ball, move your foot forward and back. As you move your foot backward, the top of it should drop down over the top of the ball a little bit. As you move forward over the ball, your heel should press down more fully. Keep your ankle flexible and notice the response in your hip and knee. You may notice that your knee or hip wants

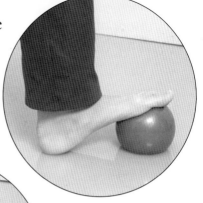

to clench. Feel the weight of those parts of the body, as much as you can. The muscles in them will still need to engage in order to keep your foot pressing into the ball, but you may find yourself using new muscles to do this. You may also find that you do not need to use very much force from your hip. Do this for 2 to 3 minutes.

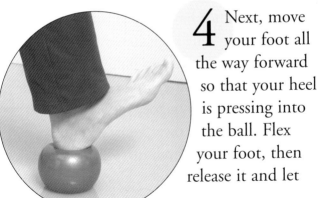

4 Next, move your foot all the way forward so that your heel is pressing into the ball. Flex your foot, then release it and let

it drape over the ball. Do this 3 times. Then pull it all the way back so that your toes are flexed and pressing into the ball. Move the toes left to right, very slowly, 3 or 4 times, or more if you have the time. Remember to breathe.

5 If you do not have very stiff feet, try this: Raise your knee straight up as though there were a string pulling it from the ceiling, until your calf dangles from your knee. Then move your toes forward and back over the ball. Lower your knee back down and drape the arch of your foot over the ball for 2 to 3 minutes. Does your hip

feel different than when you started? Feel the foot rest for a bit. Enjoy your breath. Please note that

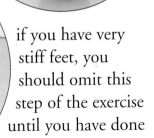

if you have very stiff feet, you should omit this step of the exercise until you have done the others to make them more limber. If you do this step with very stiff feet, you are at risk for a foot cramp.

6 Take your foot off the ball and compare your legs. Does the foot that was on the ball rest more firmly on the floor? Do more parts of it touch the floor? Does your thigh sink more into the chair? Are you breathing? Make the "S" sound.

7 Finish by stretching your leg out in front of you, leading with your foot and letting your leg follow. (If you are on an airplane you may not be able to stretch your

leg all the way.
Straighten it as
far as it will go.)
Flex your foot
several times.
Make the "S"
sound.

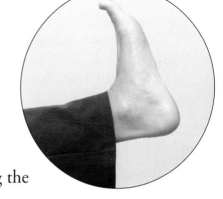

8 Repeat using the other foot.

9 If space permits, do a Seated Body Hang Over (page 118).

Exercise Six

- **Standing Up and Down on Toes (Whole Body Move)**
- **improves muscle tone; strengthens ankles and feet; supports lower back**

1 Stand up. Place your feet hip's width apart. Don't worry about how your toes are facing; do what comes naturally.

2 Support yourself against the wall (or a chair) for balance and push up onto the balls of your feet, then come back down to standing. Breathe. Do this several times.

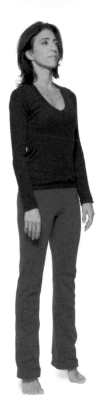

Remember that this is a Whole Body Move, not just a foot exercise. You should not let your body collapse down into your feet and expect your feet to do all the work. Let your whole body move itself upward and then press the balls of your feet against the floor. You should be pushing down against the floor and lifting your body up at the same time.

CHAPTER NINE

Ribs

The muscles around your ribcage may be some of the tightest in your body. It's a forgotten area. People tend to keep track of areas that get fat—the waistline, the thighs, even the upper arms—or of areas that are most susceptible to injury—the knees, the back, the shoulders. Ribs, though they tend not to get fatty and tend not to be a source of pain, are an important part of the healthy functioning of your body. Half of your spine is connected to your ribs, and a flexible ribcage is essential to your breathing. Your ribs can be the source of fatigue, poor posture, neck and shoulder problems, lower back pain, and disc problems. Keep your ribs flexible, however, and you'll find that you have more energy, better breathing and posture, and that it's easier to keep your back feeling good.

Exercise One

- **Ribs on the Ball Lying Down**
- **improves posture; dramatically improves breathing; eases shoulder tension and back pain**

This is an excellent ball placement to do while in bed.

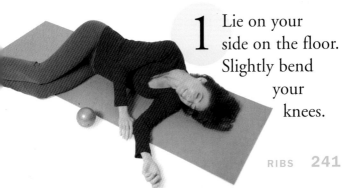

1 Lie on your side on the floor. Slightly bend your knees.

Your spine should be in a relatively straight line. Most people lie on their sides the same way they stand; their heads are often hunched in front of their ribcages.

2 Place the ball under the side of your ribs. Roll back a little, then roll your ribcage up onto the ball. Focus on initiating the movement from your ribcage itself, not from surrounding muscles, such as those in your neck.

Are you hunching over? Feel the weight of your ribcage on the ball and allow your head to roll back, elongating your spine. You'll feel more open, and you'll notice that the back of your skull rather than your forehead or cheek is resting on the floor.

3 Breathe and give in to the weight of your body. Try to avoid stiffening your

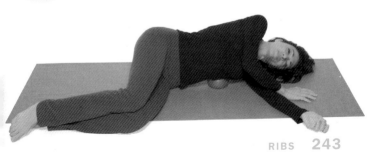

bottom shoulder. Let your weight disperse throughout your side rather than letting one body part, like your shoulder, hold your body in position.

4 Rest your top hand on the floor in front of you, with your elbow bent. Your upper arm should be resting against your chest. While resting your weight on

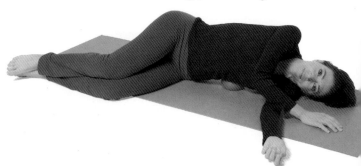

the ball, slowly move your elbow away from your body, allowing your shoulder to rotate. Then release your upper arm back toward your body. Do this 2 or 3 times. Make the "S" sound. Do you notice any changes in your shoulder?

5 Take the ball away and rest on the floor for a few minutes. Do you notice any

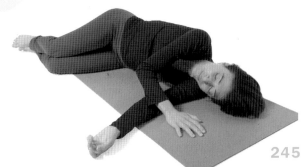

changes in the way you rest on the floor and in your breathing?

6 Repeat on both sides and, if you like, finish with the ball between your shoulder blades (see page 157).

Realize that your muscles have an incredible range of strength. Many people seem to believe that their muscles have only two settings: clenched and limp. Try to distinguish the difference between stiffening your muscles and working those muscles in a new way.

Exercise Two

- **Whole Body Twist (Whole Body Move)**
- **keeps the ribs flexible; improves breathing and muscle tone throughout the body; eases neck and shoulder tension; trims the waistline**

Remember to breathe during this exercise. You need to breathe for all the moves in the book (and for the best results in your life in general), but it's even more important here. You'll receive no benefits at all if you start to hold your breath.

1 Lie with your back on the floor. Bend your knees and rest your feet on the floor.

2 Move both legs to your left side and rest on the side of your left hip. Use gravity to let your body's weight pull your right side into the floor. Breathe.

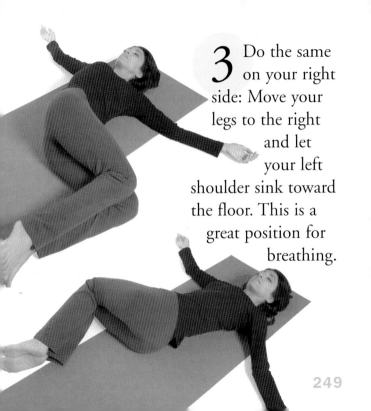

3 Do the same on your right side: Move your legs to the right and let your left shoulder sink toward the floor. This is a great position for breathing.

4 Finish lying on your back with your legs stretched out and notice how your body rests on the floor. Do you feel more of the back of your ribcage touching the floor than usual? Does your breathing reach more parts of your body?

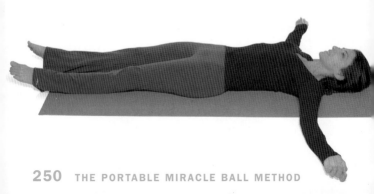

Exercise Three

- **Ribs on the Ball Seated**
- **corrects hunching; thins waistline; improves breathing**

Ribs on the Ball Seated is similar to Back on Ball Seated (page 99). It's perfect for airplanes, especially if there is an empty seat next to you; trains, where seats are usually wider than on airplanes; and desk chairs.

1 Place the ball in the middle of the back of your rib cage. Make the "S" sound and lean back against the ball. Can you feel

your breathing in your back muscles?

2 Slowly reach your hands up toward the ceiling. Keep the connection to the ball. This prevents stiff shoulders and engages stiff back muscles. Move your hands down to rest behind the back of your head, with your elbows pointing outward.

Breathe. Reach hands upward, bring them down. Repeat 2 or 3 times.

3 Gently reach your hands upward, one at a time. Notice the slight shifting of the ribcage as you alternate reaching on each side. Repeat alternate reaching 2 or 3 times. Breathe and feel the connection between your ribs and the ball.

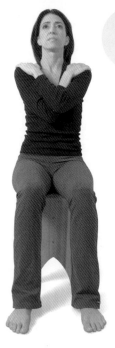

4 Bring your hands down and rest your left hand on your right shoulder, and your right hand on your left shoulder. With your arms crossed against your chest, feel the weight of your head bending forward. Allow your ribcage to round forward as your back presses against the ball. Make sure your spine is bending, not just your neck. Rest here for several seconds or as long as it's comfortable.

5 Press your ribs into the ball and come back up to a sitting position. Make sure you initiate the movement where your body connects with the ball.

6 Remove the ball, let your ribcage press against the chair. Has anything changed in your body? Is your ribcage resting differently? How is your breathing? Make the "S" sound.

- **Standing Rib Stretch and Arch (Whole Body Move)**
- **improves breathing; thins waistline; loosens neck and shoulders; relieves back tension; improves posture**

1 Stand upright with your feet hips' width apart. If you like, you may move your feet slightly more than hips' width apart, which will help you keep your balance.

2 Slowly let your body bend to the right and feel the space between your ribcage and hip open up. Don't force your body

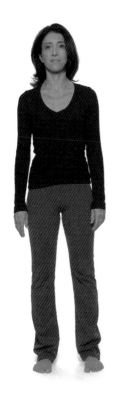

into a bend by lurching over using your back or other muscles. You should feel that the weight of your right arm is what is gently pulling your body toward the floor. Rest here for a few minutes. Make sure you are breathing.

Remember that this is a Whole Body Move, so your whole body should be participating. You should

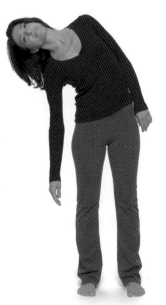

feel that your feet are pressing into the floor to create a stable base. Your legs will make an adjustment to compensate for the shift in weight, and your head should give in to gravity, stretching you from neck to waist. Allow every part of your body to make adjustments as you lean over.

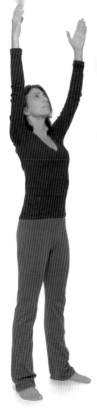

3 Return to standing. Remember to breathe. Repeat on the left side.

4 Create a ribcage arch by reaching your hands up toward the ceiling. Feel how your arms connect deep into the back of your ribcage. Lift your ribcage up and bring your arms to the back of your head. Cradle the back of your head in your hands and lift your sternum up to the ceiling, arching

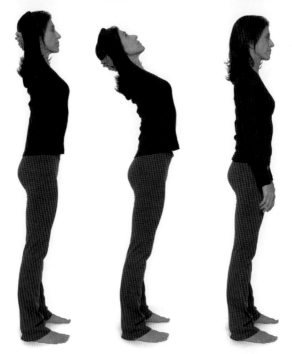

your ribcage slightly. Breathe. Bring your arms down to hang by your sides and let your ribcage soften. Do not force yourself in this position; arch only as far as is comfortable. A little arch goes a long way. Repeat this arch 3 times.

CHAPTER TEN

On The Move:
Your Conditions and
Their Prescriptions

My method is very different from traditional exercise, which targets body parts one at a time. The Miracle Ball Method uses your nervous system to connect each body part, which is the way the body naturally works. When your body is working properly, every part supports the next part, and the movements all work in relation to each other, not in isolation. This is all to say that if you do any breathing exercise with any move in this book, you will likely get relief from whatever ails you. You might be surprised to find that putting the ball under your knee will eventually bring, say, headache relief. But, indeed, it will.

My thirty years of experience with the balls have taught me, however, that there are some tried-and-true combinations of moves that work well to target certain complaints. Here are some of the most common conditions and the moves that I've found work best to address them.

Jet Lag

Keep the ball by your bed. If you wake up in the middle of the night or have difficulty sleeping, do Head on the Ball Lying Down (page 131) along with Open Mouth Breathing (page 59). This will soothe you and help release the tensions of travel. It may also help put you to sleep; if it doesn't it should ensure that when you wake up, you'll adjust more easily to a new schedule because a lot of tension will have been released.

If you find that a wall of fatigue hits you in the middle of the day, you need energy. Do Raising Your Hands (page 198) several times, then follow with the "S" sound or Open Mouth Breathing (page 59). Raising Your Hands lifts your ribcage from your diaphragm and makes the muscles around the ribcage more supple. This makes breathing easier, and easier breathing will restore your energy.

Motion Sickness

Motion sickness increases muscle tension all over your body, especially in your stomach when you start to feel nauseous. Open your mouth, soften your jaw, and exhale. Do Open Mouth Breathing (page 59) in order to stop clenching your body and holding your breath. It's all about trying to be as relaxed as possible. Put the ball under the back of your neck if you can (page 146), and try to let your whole body drape over it. These moves may prevent motion sickness from becoming worse.

Laptop/Briefcase Shoulder

Do Shoulder on the Ball (page 167) if you are forced to stay in your seat. Remember to breathe. The stiffness is largely a result of the awkward and prolonged way you hold your muscles, so you must breathe to restore feeling. Try tapping the area as well (page 65). If you don't have space to lie down, do Wrist on the Ball Seated (page 188).

Tension Headaches

Neck muscles get stiff, blood vessels constrict, and the pain makes us stop breathing, which causes even more tension.

Pick a breathing exercise and do it (pages 49–73). Then place the ball behind your neck (page 146) and breathe. Any one of the Back on the Ball exercises (pages 80–107) are also good for the sense of relaxation they bring. But breathing is the key here.

Hangover

Start in bed with Head on the Ball Lying Down (page 131) or do any other ball placement that stimulates breathing. Next, come to a seated position and do the Seated Body Hang Over (page 118). It's uncomfortable at first, but take it slowly.

Do it several times, making sure to breathe, and notice changes in between moves. Finish lying down with Back on the Ball (page 80) and let your hip joints release.

Fatigue

If you are extremely tired and need to restore energy quickly, do Raising Your Hands (page 198), Open Mouth Breathing (page 59), and Standing Body Hang Over (page 108). If you are seated, do Back on the Ball Seated (page 99).

If you are extremely tired before bed, do Calves on the Stool Lying Down, (page

92) and do your favorite breathing exercise (pages 49–73) to relax your muscles.

Stiffness

To alleviate stiffness, do the Portable Prevention Prescription (page 43), which bends your key joints to restore flexibility.

Carpal Tunnel Syndrome

Do exercises in the Wrists and Hands chapter (pages 175–200), as well as the shoulder exercises (pages 155–171), and Ball Between the Shoulder Blades Lying Down (page 157). Carpal tunnel pain is felt in the wrists and hands, but it may originate more from stiffness in the upper back between the shoulder blades. Do not overlook shoulder and upper back exercises if you are seeking relief.

Anxiety

Most people with anxiety are chronic overbreathers. They breathe in but forget to breathe out. Remember to exhale. The best breathing exercise for anxiety is Exhaling through the Straw (page 63). The "S" sound is excellent, too (page 53). Any comfortable ball exercise that helps you feel your weight and stop holding your muscles will help your breathing and help you release your overstressed muscles. I usually recommend Neck on the Ball (page 146) and Back on the Ball (pages 80 and 99). These are so relaxing that they take many people out of their thinking bodies and into their feeling bodies, which is the best way to prevent the rush of thoughts that can overwhelm us and fuel the cycle of anxiety.

Back Pain

If you have chronic lower back pain, you must breathe and reconnect with your leg joints. Any of the breathing exercises will help (pages 49–73). The best hip joint exercises are Calves on the Stool Lying Down (page 92), Seated Body Hang Over (page 118), Back on the Ball Lying Down (page 80), and Back on the Ball Seated (page 99).

If you are someone who experiences sudden back spasms and get one while traveling, try the following things as emergency treatments. First, make sure you don't start holding your breath. You must breathe in order to ensure that it doesn't get worse. Then, if you are standing and are able, bend your knees (page 120). This will relieve the pressure from your lower back. Do this slowly several times. If you can, lie on your side and do Ball between the Knees (page 212). Some people in back spasm cannot lift their legs, but if you can, try Calves on the Stool Lying Down (page 92).

Sciatica

Notice that the muscles on the side of your body where you experience pain are much tighter than those on the other side. Your goal is to loosen them. Try Hamstring Release Seated (page 223) or Standing Body Hang Over (page 108), if you can; if you can't, try Seated Body Hang Over (page 118). Calves on the Stool Lying Down (page 92) and Hamstring Release Lying Down (page 205) are also excellent for relieving sciatic pain.

Frozen Shoulder

Do Elbow on the Ball (page 184), Ball Between the Shoulder Blades (page 157), and Ribs on the Ball Seated (page 251). Make sure you are not holding your breath and do your favorite breathing exercise (pages 49–73).

Neck Pain

If you are prone to neck pain, try your first exercise of the day in bed with the ball under the back of your head (page 131). Do Open Mouth Breathing (page 59) and Head and Neck Turns (page 150).

TMJ

Breathing is essential for TMJ relief. I recommend Open Mouth Breathing (page 59), as well as Head and Neck Turns (page 150) and Face on the Ball (page 136).

Menstrual Cramps

Do Calves on the Stool Lying Down (page 92), which allows the pelvis to rest in line with your spine so that all of your internal organs rest back into your pelvis, rather than spilling forward and pressing on your belly. This enables the circulation to ease up the cramp. Do the "S" sound while you do this to ensure that you are not holding your breath.

Knee Pain

Do Calves on the Stool Lying Down (page 92), Back on the Ball (page 80), and Hamstring Release Lying Down (page 205). Standing Body Hang Over (page 108) is also excellent for relieving tight hamstrings, which can exacerbate knee pain. Just make sure not to lock your knees.

Prenatal Care

In the first trimester, Calves on the Stool Lying Down (page 92) is great for relieving lower back ache, and it is also relaxing and toning. As the pregnancy progresses, Raising Your Hands (page 198) is ideal for lifting the ribcage off the stomach. Throughout the whole nine months, especially at the end when there may be hip pain, do Ball Between the Knees Lying on Side (page 212).

Appendix by Situation

Seated Moves

Standing Moves

Lying Down Moves

Index

About the Author

Elaine Petrone developed her method of stress and pain reduction from her own experiences with chronic pain. Ms. Petrone is the author of *The Miracle Ball Method* and she has also written for and been featured in a variety of magazines, including *Fitness, Vogue, Woman's Day, Glamour, Redbook, Self, American Spa, Elle, Town & Country,* and *Harper's Bazaar.* Ms. Petrone teaches her method in hospitals, and is developing a national certification program for instructors. She can be reached at elaine@elainepetrone.com.

Acknowledgments

Many people contributed to this book coming into print.

My students have made me a better teacher and have pushed me to develop new solutions to their problems.

Thanks to the whole team at Workman Publishing Company, including Peter Workman, Suzie Bolotin, Paul Hanson, Cassie Murdoch, Doug Wolff, Page Edmunds, James Wehrle, Jenny Mandel, Kim Hicks, and Paul Gamarello. Special thanks to Jennifer Griffin, whose continued support and belief in me (as well as writing skills) have made it possible for me to keep spreading the benefits of my method. Thanks to Bob Silverstein for introducing me to Workman.

Thanks to the team at Stanford Hospital and the Health and Fitness Institute, especially Jinger Berry for her patience and support.

Finally, thanks to my children who have challenged and encouraged me throughout this whole process.